Single Scull Rowing for Beginners

A.L. Jenkins and Peinert Boatworks

Copyright © 2017 A L Jenkins

All rights reserved

1-945378-02-6

978-1-945378-02-7

www.JackWalkerPress.com

With thanks

Peinert Boat Works provided instructions and the very boats that helped launch many into the sport of sculling. They also permitted use of their *Primer On How To Scull* for use in this expanded guide. Their enthusiasm and service to rowers has provided many with a lifelong sport that supports fitness and fun.

peinert.com
Paul Milde, owner
508-758-3020
46 Marion Road (Route 6)
P.O. Box 1029
Mattapoisett, MA 02739
Email: info@sculling.com

CONTENTS

ACKNOWLEDGMENTS vii

1 Let's Begin... 1

2 Carrying the Equipment and Getting In and Out of the Boat 5

3 Rowing and turning 11

4 Problems you may encounter and how to correct them 23

5 Glossary of Terms 27

6 A Brief History of the Sport of Rowing 29

7 Health Benefits of Rowing 35

8 Additional Resources 41

ABOUT THE AUTHORS 43

ACKNOWLEDGMENTS

Thanks to all who preserve nature and clean water ways.

1

Let's Begin

Welcome to the sport of rowing, also known as sculling. This is one of the most rewarding and enjoyable of all water sports, as well as being a complete exercise and ,historically, an efficient means of transportation. However, like any new activity, a little practice is necessary at the start. Perhaps the best way to learn the sport of rowing is to get instructions from an experienced sculler. In the absence of such advice from a trusted expert, this guide should help you to get started. If you are an experienced rower, this guide will be too basic for your needs.

Peinert Boat Works of Mattapoisett, MA provided instruction for this Sculling Primer, and you'll find my personal tips and responses to using this guide as a new rower. There are no other sculls on the lake I use, so this guide, in an abbreviated form, served me well as an introductory instruction to the sport. After only a half dozen times out, I found a physical sort of Zen meditation in the coordination of body movements and the silent glide along the water. The quiet movements allow the sounds of water, ducks, and aquatic life to join me. The water seems to soak up all my errant thoughts. If you only want the exercise without the Zen—that's available to you too. Yet the Zen may sneak up on you!

You can learn this by yourself –even if you have no guide. I'm over 50 and found that after an awkward first few attempts, I could scull. I'm sculling on a long inland lake in central Arkansas and hope to be able to be active most of the year. There are no clubs nearby, and I don't transport my scull other than from my garage to the water.

This book uses spacing between paragraphs because we noticed that new users are reading and reviewing paragraphs from their boat or dock, and the spacing supports using this book as part of the action as you put the book down and seek to find your paragraph again.

The first three of the six main sections build upon each other, while the final three chapters offer ancillary information. If you are unfamiliar with sculling terms, you may wish to review the glossary in chapter three.

1. **Let's Begin**
2. **Carrying the Equipment and Getting In and Out of the Boat.**
3. **Rowing and Turning**
4. **Problems You May Encounter and How to Correct Them.**
5. **Glossary of Terms and Resources.**
6. **History of Rowing**
7. **Health Benefits**
8. **Additional Resources: Find a Rowing Club**

Because sculls are built for speed, these rowing boats are narrow and, until you become used to handling them, can tip over easily. You should start only when the water is warm and you are prepared to get wet—but you probably won't. If you can begin with an experienced mentor or rowing club, all

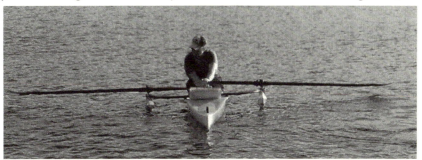

the better. You should be a swimmer and have a float device plan or wear an approved life vest. If you should capsize, do not leave the boat but rather stay with it and use the boat, cushion and/or the oars as a flotation device with which to swim to shore. It's safer to wear a life vest, but they can encumber your rowing. Consider an inflatable vest. They are expensive, generally over a hundred U.S. dollars. Totally worth it. Have a partner nearby to give you any needed assistance. Know and follow all rules associated with the body of water and community where you row.

I use a scull with pontoons that help to keep the boat stable, but I did tip it once when figuring out how to get into the scull in a non-ideal launch area. The water was warm and no problems resulted. Be prepared for this to happen to you.

Consider phones and other pocket contents, watches, slippery rocks, cold water, and how you might get to safety if you take a tumble. Be prepared.

Wear sunglasses and a hat to protect your eyes. Use sunscreen. Gloves may help your hands from getting banged up. Especially in the early stages of learning to scull, it's easy to bump the backs of your hands. I use biking gloves, but you can use more specialized gloves if you choose. Dress for the weather. When you scull, you assume responsibility for all involved risks.

You should read through the entire text first, then concentrate on the instruction section. Take your time, relax, and enjoy learning to row. Don't try to row too fast at the beginning; it will probably take a couple of outings before you feel comfortable and can fully enjoy the sport. The first time or two that you scull, you may want to practice your arm movements alone. Keep your legs extended and practice the rows. Then add and coordinate your leg movements.

2

Carrying the Equipment and Getting In and Out of the Boat

The boat is easy to carry. It can be carried by two people, one at each end, or by one person from the side, canoe-fashion. The oar blades are thin and can be broken with little difficulty, so you should always carry them with the blades in front of you to decrease the possibility of hitting anything with them. Use care in putting them down and into the boat. When leaving the dock or shore, be careful not to hit them against anything. The seat will stay in the boat when it is being carried short distances, but if you are going to transport the boat you should remove the seat. Simply pull it off the bow end of the tracks. To put the seat in the boat, set the stern pair of wheels on the tracks at the bow end. Make sure that the retaining clips on the underside of the seat are going under the flange on the track, and push the seat on towards the stern. If the boat is too heavy for you, as it was for me, you might want to consider a kayak carrier. I use bungee cords to hold the scull to a small two-wheeled kayak carrier when no one is available to help.

Because you face backwards while rowing, the bow is at your back. In a kayak, you'll face the bow, but in a scull, you face the stern. The straighter edge of the seat is parallel to the abdomen, while the curved end is parallel to the back. Pictures of the seat follow.

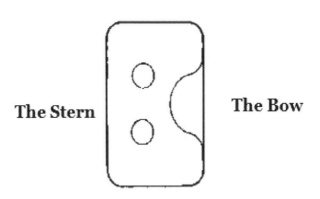

The Stern　　　　　　　　**The Bow**

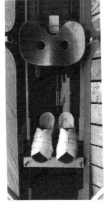

Once you have the boat, with seat, in the water, either at the dock or next to the shore, put the oars in the locks. This is done by placing the thin part of the oar shaft near the blade into the lock, then sliding the oar out into the lock until the button contacts the lock. It is easiest to push off in a boat that is parallel to a dock or the shore. One should keep the oars relatively perpendicular to the boat while embarking or disembarking, and not try to "ship" the oars as in a fixed-seat rowboat. Don't stow the paddle end of the oar on the hull of the boat.

Keep the paddles extended flat on the water/pier to add to the stability of the boat.

To get into the boat, hold both oar grips with one hand, buttons out against the locks, oar blades flat, and the oars perpendicular to the boat. Place the other hand on the convenient edge of the boat, place one foot on the non-slip surface between the tracks and step in. As you step in, the oars should be in front of your body (to the stern) and the seat should be behind (to the bow) so that you can sit. Should the seat be out of position, sit on the platform and adjust yourself onto it once in the boat. Once sitting down, place each foot in the shoes or under the respective loop on the foot-board and adjust the strap to be just snug. It is easy to do this if you bring both oar handles into your armpits; blades resting on the surface of the water, extend your arms over the handles and roll forward on the seat so that the oar handle is positioned between your thighs and arms.

If you don't have ideal conditions, you may find the need to improvise, but be warned: anytime you play fast and loose with the ideal entry conditions, your likelihood of a dunking increases. Getting wet may not be a problem but be aware that falls can be dangerous. Wet conditions, slippery rocks, fast currents and more could spell injury or worse. My only injuries have been a finger blister and sore muscles and joints.

I have added a floating platform to the end of our fixed dock. Previously, when entering the boat, our dock was often two feet above the water. Because our lake level varied so widely, my strategy would be different as the water level fluctuated. If the water was high, and approached the level of the dock, I could use a standard entry strategy with my oars perpendicular to the scull—the recommended entry position. Other times, I entered the water from a shallow shore. I'd step into the water, sit on the seat and rotate my legs into the scull.

I searched the internet for videos of entering the scull from a high dock and found a suggested maneuver, but I didn't have the dexterity to perform the suggested method. If you are fit, flexible, and have a good sense of balance, you might want to give a YouTube search a try. At the writing of this primer a helpful video was available. I searched the phrase "getting into a scull from a high dock." This instructional video advises one to bring the boat close to the dock by placing the outriggers (holds the oar locks) at the end of the dock. If you think of the boat as a giant "t," the outriggers are the short line on the letter. Pull the scull to the end of the dock until the outriggers (short line on the "t") are beyond the end of the dock. Then the boat is close enough to the dock or pier to be able to step a foot onto the platform. The rower needs to step onto the boat platform with one foot and to shift weight to sit down and place the alternate foot on the rowing platform. Then both feet need to be adjusted into the straps.

It is important to maintain control over both oar handles at all times, or you may tip over. The oar blades act as outriggers and prevent you from rolling over as long as you keep your hold on the grips. It is only when you let go of one of the oars or let it turn completely parallel to the boat hull that you are most subject to a roll over.

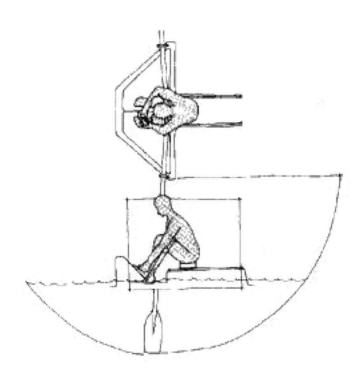

Position to adjust foot strap.

If you are embarking from the shore, you can probably just

row away, being careful not to let the oar blades hit the bottom. If you get in from a dock, you will now want to reach over with your arm, holding on to both grips with the other hand, and push yourself away as strongly as possible. This may not get you far enough off the dock to begin rowing. Lean away from the dock a little, onto the outside oar blade, and pull the inside oar carefully in towards you until you can place the blade on the edge of the dock and push away. The boats are very responsive.

To return to the dock, it is best to approach at an angle slowly. Just as the blade would hit the dock, lean away from the dock onto the outside blade. This will cause the boat to turn parallel to the dock as it comes in and will enable you to get the inside blade raised up onto the dock. You should practice this maneuver a couple of times away from the dock. If out for the first or second time, have your helper/observer pull you in with the oar once you get close enough.

Rowing with a club will likely afford you good entry conditions and helpful companions. But you can learn this on your own as a solidary sport. It's my sacred alone time—good for body and spirit.

3

Rowing and turning

There are at least two elements to sculling which are probably new to you:

1. Feathering, which is the turning flat of the oar blades as you release them from the water at the end of the stroke and the turning perpendicular again right before the catch, where you put them back in the water. Feathering makes it easier to extract the blades from the water, cuts wind resistance on the recovery, and makes it easier to row in choppy water.

On a few occasions, I've accidentally brought the paddle out of the water with the broad part parallel to the water. This action created a jarring movement that made the boat feel unstable. The skinny blade of the paddle should enter and leave the water. This will create a smooth ride.

2. The use of the sliding seat, which enables you to use your legs to propel the boat.

Let's start with a basic rest position, the most comfortable position in which to sit when not moving. Sit squarely on the seat, feet under the straps, knees down so that the backs of the calves are touching the boat, one hand on each oar with the handles just in front of the body over the thighs, oar blades flat on the water, concave side up.

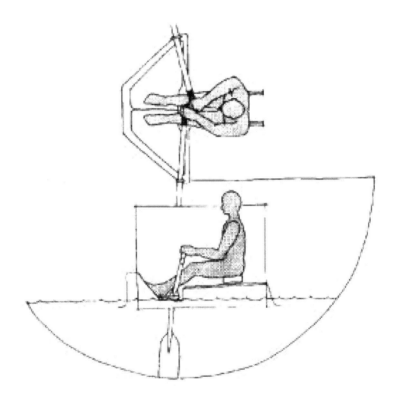

Still sitting in the rest position, place the hands on the grips so that they would be in the proper position for the drive; the blade should be floating at the surface of the water, concave side towards the stern. Your fingers should be wrapped loosely around the grip with your thumb across the end of the grip. Use the thumbs to press lightly outwards at all times so that the buttons stay in contact with the locks. Your wrist should be relatively flat. If it is particularly arched up or down, you will have trouble with the feathering and your forearm will tire quickly.

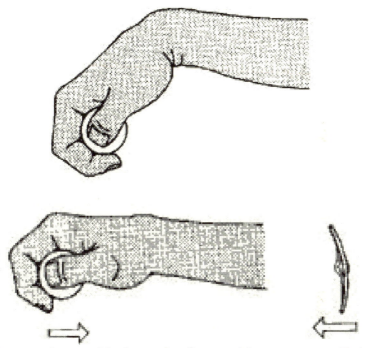

To change the oar blade to the flat position, as you will do at the finish of each stroke, one gives a relaxed twist to the grip. Drop the wrist slightly while rolling the top of the grip towards the chest, while at the same time letting the oar shaft drop flat into the oarlock and the grip roll out more under the fingers.

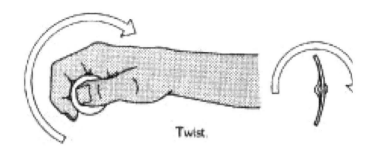

Twist.

Twist.

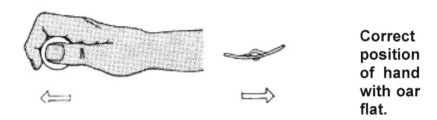

Correct position of hand with oar flat.

Actually, the blade does not quite go all the way flat; the front edge is slightly higher than the back edge to help keep it from digging into the water on the recovery.

To move the blade back to vertical, merely squeeze the fingers toward the palm, re-closing the grip and bringing the wrist back up to the flat position.

You may find it easier to determine the correct grip and hand movements for feathering by practicing for a minute or two on the shore before you step into the boat. Oar rotation is easier if you use a little grease, such as Crisco or Vaseline, on the button and sleeve of the oar where it moves in the oarlock.

You should now be sitting on the water in the rest position with some idea of how to feather. We will practice a turn and feathering at the same time. This will enable us to practice feathering with one hand at a time, while learning to turn around without tipping over.

To turn to port, your right as you sit in the boat, and practice with the left hand, start by slightly lowering the port grip with your right hand and leaning slightly towards the port (your right). You should look like the sketch:

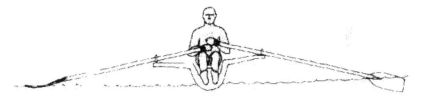

In this position you can row with your left hand without fear of interference with the other hand.

The feathering of the blade is done at the following points in the stroke: The blade is held flat and a couple of inches off the water on the recovery until just before the catch. It is returned to the vertical position in time to be placed in the water for the drive. It is held vertical through the drive (easy to do since the flat on the oar-shaft pulls into the corresponding flat surface on the oar-lock). It is turned flat as it is taken out of the water. If turned too soon, while still pulling on the oar, the blade will knife deeply into the water; if turned too late it is harder to release the blade from the water. The correct path of the blade in air and water is shown in the sketch.

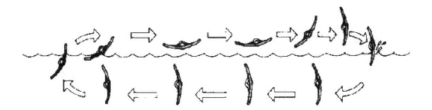

Note that the blade follows a rectangular path with rounded ends.

Now, to row. It may be easiest to start without using the sliding seat; that is, just sitting with the legs down flat and rowing with your arms and upper body swing until you get a little more used to the feathering.

You will notice that the oar handles overlap in the middle of the recovery and drive. The starboard (your left as you sit in the boat,) oarlock is set slightly higher than the port and you will want to row with the left hand slightly higher than the right, so that in the middle of the stroke the starboard grip is directly over the port grip.

To row using the sliding seat, start at the rest position, extend the arms straight towards the stern, swing your upper body over towards the stern and then roll on the seat as far towards the stern as is comfortable. Feather the blades up towards the vertical position and place them into the water as you get to your full extension.

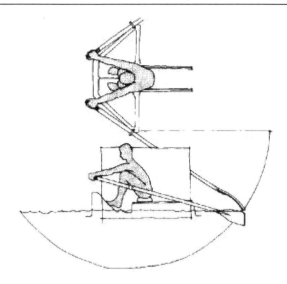

Position at the catch or beginning of the drive.

Your knees should stay close together so that they come up either under the armpit or in front of your chest.

The first half of the drive is accomplished by a push of the legs and a simultaneous swing towards the bow with the torso, keeping the arms straight.

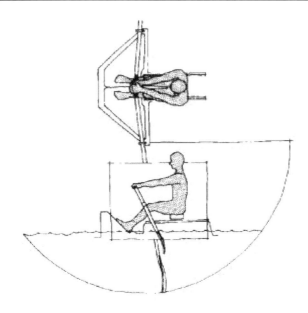

Midway through the drive.

Only when the legs are fully extended do you begin to pull in with the arms, at the same time finishing the swing of the upper body to a position about 10 degrees past the vertical.

Single Scull Rowing for Beginners

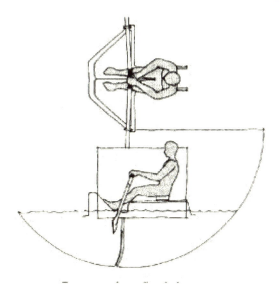

Beginning the pull with the arms.

Your elbows should be hanging down in a relaxed position so that they will pass closely by your torso as you finish the stroke.

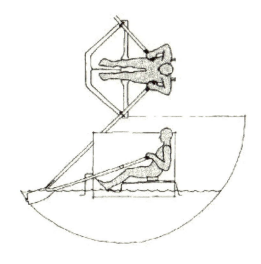

Position at the finish of the drive.

As the oars swing through so that the grips point at your sides, lightly press down on the handles and simultaneously turn the blades flat as described earlier.

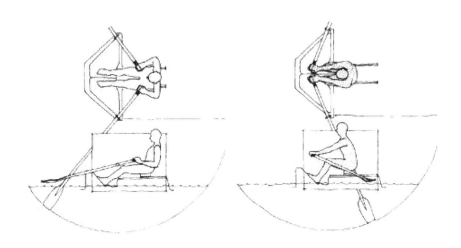

The release.　　　　　　**The recovery.**

Once the blades are out of the water at the finish, you accomplish the recovery by straightening your arms, remembering to keep the left hand over the right, and moving the grips toward the stern on a level path.

As the arms straighten, let the upper body swing over towards the stern. Once the oar handles are past your knees, begin rolling on the slide towards the stern, keeping the arms straight and the upper body reaching for the next catch. Just before getting to your full reach, turn the blades to vertical and prepare to lightly let them drop into the water.

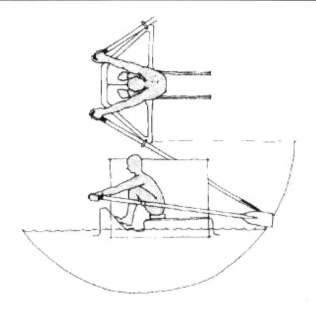

Position at the end of the recovery.

As you stop rolling on the seat and with the blades in, begin pushing off for the next drive.

It may be easier to balance at first if you let the oar blades just touch the water on the recovery, acting as outriggers. However, you will soon find that you can row more smoothly, especially in choppy water, if you keep them a couple of inches off the surface.

From the stern, two points to note:

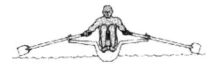

Correct, knees close together at the catch.

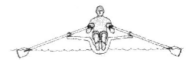

Correct, elbows close to the sides at the finish.

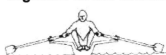

Incorrect, knees splayed.

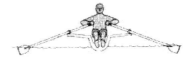

Incorrect, elbows out.

4

Problems you may encounter and how to correct them

1. It is hard to release the blades from the water at the finish.

You may have the blade too deep in the water (it should be just covered) or you may be feathering it too soon or too late. Turn the blade flat just as you release it from the water.

2. The oar handles hit my knees on the recovery.

You should keep your legs extended and knees down until your arms are fully extended and your upper body has swung over towards the stern, at which point the handles are then over your shins, clear of your knees and you can begin to roll towards the stern.

Or, you may be trying to keep the oar blades too high off the water with the handles too low. If this is the case, try keeping the oar blades only a couple of inches off the water with your hands a little higher over the knees.

Or, try raising the height of the oarlocks a little.

3. My forearms get tired.

Try a more relaxed grip on the oar handle.

Or, be sure your wrist is flat as you pull the oar through the water.

Or, be sure you have put Crisco or Vaseline on the button and sleeve to allow the oar to turn more easily in the lock as you feather.

4. The seat binds and doesn't roll well

Be sure you are sitting in the middle of the seat and not twisting as you roll back and forth, or the seat might need oil.

5. The back of the legs hit the seat rail.

Reposition the foot length so the hamstring area doesn't hit the seat rail. Or you may place a towel under your legs –as long as it doesn't become entangled in the seat rail.

6. It is hard to keep the blades from diving deep on the drive.

You are probably not turning the oar-blade all the way to vertical before putting it in the water at the catch; be sure your grip on the oar handle is relaxed and be sure the oar blade is vertical before catching the water, and relax your grip as you pull so that the flat of the oar shaft can align itself with the flat of the oarlock, which keeps the oar blade in the proper position.

7. I can't see where I'm going.

You might consider a mirror used by bikers to see behind them. They can attach to sunglasses or hats. The field of vision in these is small, but you can learn to use them to see some of the area you are rowing to. As always, use caution.

I use a bike mirror and I find even the small field of view is helpful.

8. My back gets sore.

General back health is important to rowing. Work with a healthcare professional if you have back problems. You can minimize the risk of back injuries by avoiding rowing for too long. Fatigue may engender poor posture. Rowers should aim to keep their backs gently straight with a slight C-curve. They should neither slump nor keep rigidly flat-backed.

According to *World Rowing*, biomechanical analysis in both the lab and on the water has shown that the position of the pelvis has a crucial role to play in preventing injury. Rowers "should flex through the hips, rocking the trunk forward over the 'sit bones', particularly in the transition from the drive to recovery, keeping the lower back in a fairly neutral position." When a rower is tired, he or she may move the back more instead of maintaining good hip movement. This tendency can strain or injure the back.

Take care to avoid leaning your torso too far past a 90-degree angle with the floor. This puts your back in a weak position.

9. It is hard to keep the boat level while rowing.

Be sure to keep your body balanced over the center of the boat.

Work on releasing the water smoothly at the finish so that you start the recovery on an even keel. If the oar isn't vertical as it comes out of the water, the resistance will likely cause the boat to wobble.

Be sure to keep the oar handles moving on a constant level; moving the handles up and down affects the balance of the boat.

5

Glossary of Terms

Blade: The flat part of the oar that goes into the water

Bow: The front of the boat

Button: Plastic collar on the oar shaft, located over the sleeve, and locates the oar against the oarlock when in use

Catch: The point in the stroke at which the blades are put into the water at the beginning of the drive, also the end of the recovery

Drive: That portion of the stroke when the blades are in the water and the person is pulling on the oar handles

Feathering: The act of twisting the oar to position the blade vertically for the drive and horizontally for the recovery

Grips: Rubber caps on the inboard (handle) end of the oars

Oarlock: Plastic piece that holds the oar and pivots, located on the end of the rigger

Pin: Bolt that forms the pivot for the oarlock

Port: Left side of the boat facing forward, right side as you sit to row, often marked red.

Recovery: That part of the stroke when the blades are out of the water and the person is moving towards the next drive

Release: That point at which the oars are taken out of the water at the end of the drive, also the beginning of the recovery

Rigger: Arm extending out from the side of the boat, it holds the pin and oarlock

Sculls: Another name for the oars, sculling is also another name for the act of rowing

Sleeve: Plastic tube on the oar, under the button, that protects against wear in the oarlock

Starboard: Right side of the boat facing forward, left side as you sit to row, often marked green

Stern: Back of the boat

6

A Brief History of the Sport of Rowing

Ancient and Early History

Rowing has a history as one of oldest sports traditions in the world-- nearly as long as the history of humankind. An Egyptian funerary inscription of 1430 BC celebrates the warrior Amenhotep for his skills in oarsmanship. Virgil writes about rowing as a part of the funeral games for Aeneid in the famous epic poem, *The Aeneid*, which was written between 29 and19 BC.

The sport likely grew out the skills needed to transport and commit warfare across the water. Rowing survived as a sport through the Dark and Middle Ages. During the 14th century, rowing teams raced the narrow canals in the Carnevale regattas of Italy. In England, guilds sponsored boats to compete in the Lord Mayor's Water Procession beginning in

1454. Watermen competed on the River Thames in London in the early 10th Century. The river was used in transportation of people and goods and watermen were the engines that powered this practice. Rowing in its modern form developed in England in the 1700s.

More European Rowing History

The Doggett's Coat and Badge race is the oldest rowing competition in the world. The race began in 1715 and continues every year on the Thames, "between London Bridge and Cadogan Pier (Chelsea) - the sites of the Old Swan Tavern and the Swan Inn Chelsea. Up to six young watermen will row under 11 bridges on the 4 mile 7 furlong (7,400 meter) course" according to the Doggett's Race for Coat and Badge website.

Rowing in the US and Modern Olympic Era

Rowing spread to the US. In 1762, six-oared barges raced on the Schuylkill River in Pennsylvania. Popularity of the sport continued to grow. The first US rowing club, the Detroit Boat Club, was founded in 1839.

In 1852 Harvard and Yale held the first intercollegiate sport contest in the United States. Harvard won. The annual race continues to this day.

Rowing was included in the first modern Olympics, but bad weather prevented the race. Male rowers have competed since the 1900 Paris Olympics, and women's racing was added in 1976. Paralympic Games included rowing as a competitive sport in Beijing's 2008 competition.

In 1976, rowing played a part in providing women equal access to school sports.

Title IX of the Education Amendments Act of 1972 is a federal law that states:

No person in the United States shall, on the basis of sex, be excluded from participation in, be denied the benefits of, or be subjected to discrimination under any education program or activity receiving Federal financial assistance.

Although Title IX had been passed in 1972, the Yale woman's rowing team was fed up with what they called less than human treatment. Their shells were antiquated, their annual funding was dismal, and they had no showers. After practice, the men took warm showers, while the women sat on a cold bus waiting. They often practiced in winter and were wet from sweat on the inside of their clothing, and ice and icy water on the outside of their clothing. One of the rowers came down with pneumonia. The athletic department ignored the rower's pleas, so the women carried out a protest. They invited a New York Times stringer and prepared for the protest by writing a statement and writing on each other's backs and sternums. They wrote the word "TITLE IX" or" IX."

The athletes walked into the Athletic department director's office, removed their clothes, and read their "Declaration of Accountability."

> *These are the bodies Yale is exploiting. We have come here today to make clear how unprotected we are, to show graphically what we are being exposed to ... We are not just healthy young things in blue and white uniforms who perform feats of strength for Yale in the nice spring weather; we are not just statistics on your win column. We're human and being treated as less than such.*
>
> —Part of the statement read by Chris Ernst on behalf of 1976 Yale women's crew.

The athletes gained publicity, vast public support, and their showers. More importantly, those schools across the nation that did not take title IX seriously were prodded to change policies to meet their legal obligation to women's sports.

Endnotes Sources for Chapter 6

"Rowing History-Home." Rowing History-Home. Accessed December 06, 2016. http://www.rowinghistory.net/.

"The History of Rowing." The History of Rowing. Accessed December 06, 2016. http://www.athleticscholarships.net/history-rowing.htm.

Wulf, Steve. "ESPN The Magazine -- The 1976 Protest That Helped Define Title IX Movement." EspnW. July 14, 2012. Accessed December 06, 2016. http://www.espn.com/espnw/title-ix/article/7985418/espn-magazine-1976-protest-helped-define-title-ix-movement.

7

Health Benefits of Rowing

Find an exercise you like and you are likely to improve your quality of life as well as your lifespan. If you love rowing, you are lucky because rowing tends to be high in benefits and low in joint impact and injuries. The benefits are so significant that this is a sport you should try if you have access to equipment and a place to row. Using a rowing machine (ergometer) is becoming a hot new sport. Some say the rowing is the new spinning—but rowing is even better and provides a more balanced full-body workout. If you love the water and nature, gliding across a lake or river or even calm ocean waters can be both calming and motivating. Once the technique of rowing becomes habit, the movements can build power and strength to your cardiovascular system and muscle groups. Rowers are responsible to engage in physical activity that is appropriate to their health status under the supervision of a health care professional.

Get rid of extra fat

Rowing is predominately an aerobic sport. According to fitness trainer Aamir Becic, most rowers can easily burn up to 600 calories an hour, while competitive rowers expend almost twice the number of calories on a 2,000-meter course as a runner in a 3,000-meter steeplechase. Rowing can promote a healthy balance of fat to muscle in disciplined rowers.

Tone everywhere

Rowing, when done correctly, works the back, hamstrings, gluteal muscles, biceps, and core. It utilizes more body parts than most cardiovascular gym equipment. People of many different fitness levels can approach the sport. Rowing just might be the most efficient exercise ever. "With each stroke, pretty much every part of the body is used," says Stella Lucia Volpe, an exercise physiologist and professor of nutrition sciences at Drexel University in Philadelphia and an avid rower. And it may let you skip crunches—for good. "A big part of rowing is core strength," she adds. "People think it's all arms, but rowing is much more legs and core."

As quadriceps become stronger, activities and exercises such as walking, jogging, lunges and squats can be done more efficiently.

Be good to your cardio-respiratory system

Cardiovascular training involves any activity that requires the use of the large muscle groups of the body in a regular and uninterrupted manner. Rowing is one of the few non-weight bearing sports that exercises all the major muscle groups.

Rowing at a steady state for only 30 minutes can enhance the lungs' ability to provide oxygen to the blood. Rowing can be done every day, or combined with other activities on non-rowing days for terrific cross training. Thirty minutes of daily aerobic activity is linked to better heart health. Interval training with high intensity spurts is also shown to be effective in improving health outcomes.

"Rowing is a full-body exercise, and it keeps the heart rate elevated," says Garrett Roberts, an exercise physiologist and personal trainer who founded GoRow Studios in Hoboken, New Jersey. "But then it is leg press after leg press and row after row, so there's a huge strength-training component to it too." Which is why you'll get a svelte physique faster. "Rowing burns two to three times the amount of calories of Spinning," explains Roberts. "Unlike a bike, which only has resistance in one direction, rowing has resistance in both directions—forward and back—making you much stronger and increasing the rate at which you burn calories."

Row away stress

The consistent and rhythmic activity associated with rowing, combined with being outdoors on the water, has an unparalleled impact on reducing stress. For some the effect can be similar to stationary or walking meditation. Those who participate in meditative activities often have an increased feeling of well-being and describe a better quality of life.

Enjoy low impact with high results

Both competitive and recreational rowing are unique in comparison to most sports because they exercise all of your major muscle groups. Everything from your legs, back and arms are engaged while rowing. Rowing is a low-impact sport. When executed properly, the rowing stroke is a fairly safe motion, providing little room for the serious injury often found in contact and high-impact sports.

Improve mobility

Rowing exercises and conditions many different muscles and joints without significant stress or risk of injury. This makes rowing ideal for many with arthritis or osteoporosis. The muscles and joints experience a wide range of movement during rowing, which can minimize stiffness and increase flexibility. Most people will feel muscles and joints loosen up after 20 to 30 minutes of rowing at a moderate pace.

Stabilize the body

Rowing in a boat requires the stabilizer and neutralizer muscles to fire up. A strong core can prevent falls. Those same muscles might help to avoid a fall or protect the back when lifting a child or a heavy object.

Endnote sources for Chapter Seven

Catanese, Nicole. "Rowing Is The New Spinning." Harper's BAZAAR. September 16, 2014. Accessed December 14, 2016. http://www.harpersbazaar.com/beauty/diet-fitness/advice/a3549/rowing-fitness-trend-1014/ 1.3k.

"Top 10 Health Benefits of Rowing • Health Fitness Revolution." Health Fitness Revolution. April 7, 2015. Accessed December 14, 2016. http://www.healthfitnessrevolution.com/top-10-health-benefits-rowing/.

8

Additional Resources

Even if your rowing aspirations were solitary, you might also enjoy the competition, support, and camaraderie offered in a club.

Rowing Clubs

Find a rowing club in Australia

> http://www.rowingaustralia.com.au/

Find a rowing club in Europe

> http://www.rowinglinks.com/europe/clubs/

Find a rowing club in South Africa

> http://www.rowsa.co.za/Venues

Find a rowing club in the UK

> https://www.britishrowing.org

Find a rowing club in the USA

> http://www.usrowing.org

ABOUT THE AUTHORS

A.L Jenkins is the award-winning author of *Every Natural Fact: Five Seasons of Open-Air Parenting*. She writes nature, science, health, and parenting books under the name Amy Lou Jenkins. She also writes for children under the name Lou Jenkins. Contact her through Jack Walker Press.

www.JackWalkerPress.com

PEINERT Boatworks provided the instructional part of this book and many of the illustrations.

Peinert boats bring elite performance and light weight to durable, affordable shells.

Peinert single sculls are moderately priced boats built with the best materials to have the speed and feel of an elite boat while being durable and easy to row.

http://peinert.com/

508-758-3020
46 Marion Road (Route 6)
P.O.Box 1029
Mattapoisett, MA 02739 Email: info@sculling.com

Made in the USA
Middletown, DE
02 July 2023